DIABETES-FRIENDLY KIDNEY MEALS

Delicious and Nutritious Recipes to Manage Your Health

Dr Lily Morgan

COPYRIGHT PAGE

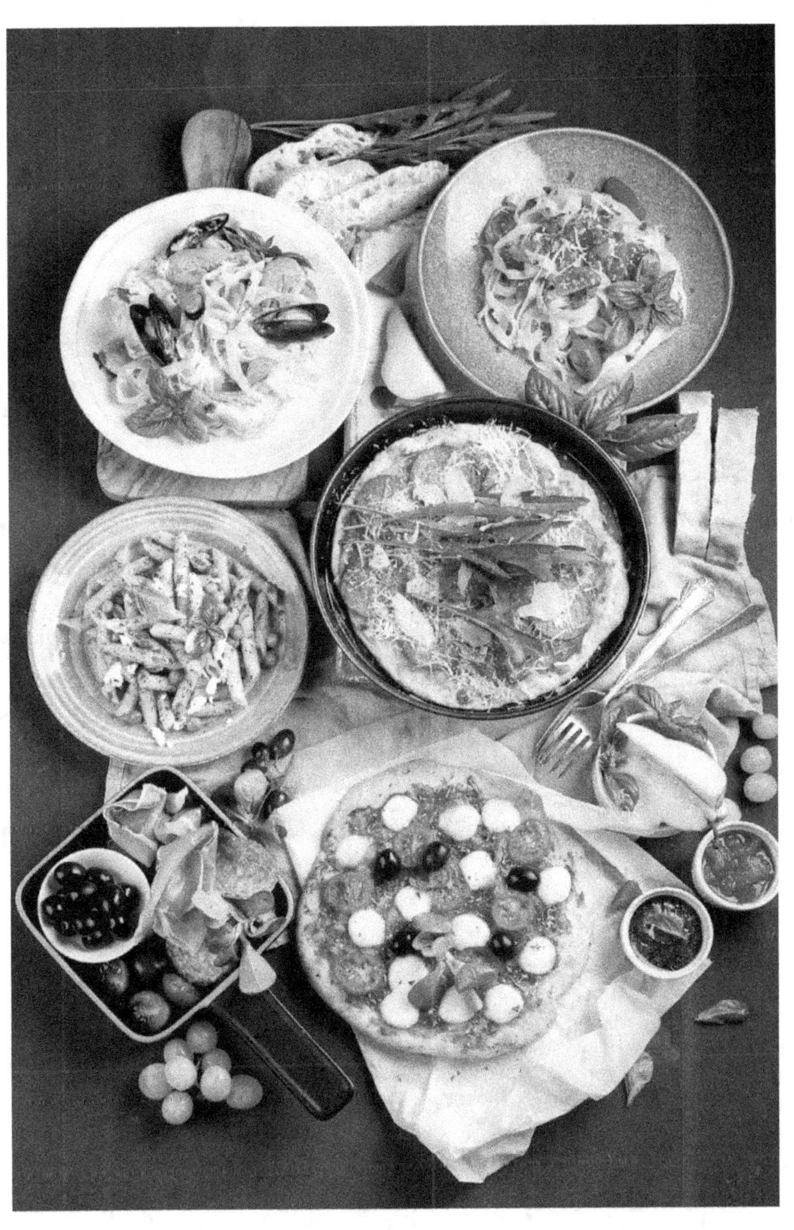

TABLE OF CONTENTS

Chapter 3: Lunch Recipes 37

Chapter 4: Dinner Recipes 54

Chapter 5: Snacks and Appetizers 74

Chapter 6: Desserts 86

CONCLUSION 102

INTRODUCTION

Understanding the intricate relationship between Diabetes and Kidney Health is paramount for anyone facing these intertwined health challenges. These two conditions often coexist and require a delicate balance to manage effectively.

Diabetes, characterized by high blood sugar levels, can take a toll on the kidneys over time. The kidneys play a pivotal role in regulating blood sugar and filtering waste products. When diabetes is uncontrolled, it can lead to kidney damage, a condition known as diabetic nephropathy. This underscores the significance of maintaining optimal blood sugar levels to protect kidney health.

Nutrition, therefore, becomes the cornerstone in managing these conditions. A well-planned, diabetes-friendly diet not only helps control blood sugar but also eases the burden on the kidneys. It's essential to strike a balance between carbohydrates, proteins, and fats, taking into account the unique needs of both diabetes and kidney health.

Low-sodium choices are key in preserving kidney function. Excess sodium can lead to fluid retention and high blood pressure, both of which are detrimental to the kidneys. A diet rich in fruits and vegetables, while low in processed foods, can be instrumental in reducing sodium intake.

Managing carbohydrates is another crucial aspect. Carbohydrates directly affect blood sugar levels, and people with diabetes must be mindful of their carbohydrate intake. For those with kidney issues, it's important to select carbohydrates that are lower in phosphorus, as high phosphorus levels can be harmful to the kidneys.

Proteins, while essential for the body, can be taxing on the kidneys if consumed in excess. Individuals with both diabetes and kidney conditions should focus on lean protein sources and monitor their intake.

In essence, nutrition becomes a dual strategy in managing diabetes and kidney health. It's about maintaining stable blood sugar levels to protect the kidneys and making dietary choices that don't overburden these vital organs. This intricate dance of balancing nutrition and health is at the heart of successfully managing these interconnected conditions.

Chapter 1: 30 Day Meal Plan

Week 1:

Day 1:

- Breakfast: Vegetable Omelette
- Lunch: Grilled Chicken Salad
- Dinner: Baked Herb-Crusted Cod
- Snacks: Roasted Almonds
- Dessert: Berry Parfait

Day 2:

- Breakfast: Cinnamon Oatmeal
- Lunch: Lentil and Vegetable Soup
- Dinner: Chicken and Veggie Skewers
- Snacks: Guacamole and Veggie Sticks
- Dessert: Dark Chocolate-Dipped Strawberries

Day 3:

- Breakfast: Greek Yogurt Parfait
- Lunch: Turkey and Avocado Wrap
- Dinner: Quinoa-Stuffed Bell Peppers

- Snacks: Hummus with Whole Wheat Pita
- Dessert: Baked Apples with Cinnamon

Day 4:

- Breakfast: Spinach and Mushroom Frittata
- Lunch: Quinoa and Black Bean Bowl
- Dinner: Beef and Vegetable Stir-Fry
- Snacks: Cucumber Slices with Tzatziki
- Dessert: Greek Yogurt Cheesecake

Day 5:

- Breakfast: Avocado Toast
- Lunch: Salmon with Asparagus
- Dinner: Garlic and Herb Shrimp
- Snacks: Deviled Eggs
- Dessert: Sugar-Free Pudding

Day 6:

- Breakfast: Blueberry Quinoa Porridge
- Lunch: Tofu Stir-Fry
- Dinner: Spinach and Mushroom Stuffed Chicken
- Snacks: Edamame

* Dessert: Almond Flour Brownies

Day 7:

* Breakfast: Breakfast Burrito
* Lunch: Caprese Salad
* Dinner: Lemon-Dill Salmon
* Snacks: Cheese and Whole Wheat Crackers
* Dessert: Chia Seed Chocolate Pudding

Week 2:

Day 8:

* Breakfast: Smoothie Bowl
* Lunch: Minestrone Soup
* Dinner: Vegetable Curry
* Snacks: Greek Yogurt with Berries
* Dessert: Mixed Berry Sorbet

Day 9:

* Breakfast: Chia Seed Pudding
* Lunch: Chickpea and Spinach Salad
* Dinner: Mushroom and Lentil Shepherd's Pie
* Snacks: Mixed Nuts

- Dessert: Banana Nut Muffins

Day 10:

- Breakfast: Whole Wheat Pancakes
- Lunch: Veggie and Hummus Wrap
- Dinner: Spaghetti Squash with Turkey Meatballs
- Snacks: Sliced Bell Peppers with Salsa
- Dessert: Oatmeal Raisin Cookies

Day 11:

- Breakfast: Breakfast Casserole
- Lunch: Teriyaki Chicken Bowl
- Dinner: Tofu and Vegetable Stir-Fry
- Snacks: Avocado Salsa
- Dessert: Avocado Chocolate Mousse

Day 12:

- Breakfast: Berry Protein Smoothie
- Lunch: Zucchini Noodles with Pesto
- Dinner: Pork Tenderloin with Roasted Veggies
- Snacks: Caprese Skewers
- Dessert: Pumpkin Pie Chia Pudding

Day 13:

- Breakfast: Scrambled Tofu
- Lunch: Turkey and Cranberry Quinoa Salad
- Dinner: Cilantro-Lime Black Bean Salad
- Snacks: Baked Sweet Potato Fries
- Dessert: Peach Cobbler

Day 14:

- Breakfast: Nut Butter and Banana Toast
- Lunch: Tuna Salad Lettuce Wraps
- Dinner: Roasted Garlic and Rosemary Chicken
- Snacks: Spinach and Artichoke Dip
- Dessert: Berry Crisp

Week 3:

Day 15:

- Breakfast: Rice Pudding with Stevia
- Lunch: Spicy Cauliflower Soup
- Dinner: Teriyaki Portobello Mushrooms
- Snacks: Stuffed Mushrooms
- Dessert: Tiramisu Cups

Day 16:

- Breakfast: Tofu and Vegetable Stir-Fry
- Lunch: Greek Quinoa Salad
- Dinner: Baked Eggplant Parmesan
- Snacks: Quinoa Salad Cups
- Dessert: Orange Sorbet

Day 17:

- Breakfast: Sweet Potato Hash
- Lunch: Eggplant and Tomato Stack
- Dinner: Thai Red Curry with Tofu
- Snacks: Chicken Lettuce Wraps
- Dessert: Chocolate Protein Balls

Day 18:

- Breakfast: Egg and Spinach Breakfast Quesadilla
- Lunch: Shrimp and Broccoli Stir-Fry
- Dinner: Sweet Potato and Chickpea Tagine
- Snacks: Cottage Cheese with Pineapple
- Dessert: Baked Apples with Cinnamon

Day 19:

- Breakfast: Quinoa and Fruit Bowl
- Lunch: Greek Yogurt Parfait
- Dinner: Grilled Chicken Salad
- Snacks: Roasted Almonds
- Dessert: Dark Chocolate-Dipped Strawberries

Day 20:

- Breakfast: Avocado Toast
- Lunch: Lentil and Vegetable Soup
- Dinner: Baked Herb-Crusted Cod
- Snacks: Guacamole and Veggie Sticks
- Dessert: Berry Parfait

Day 21:

- Breakfast: Blueberry Quinoa Porridge
- Lunch: Turkey and Avocado Wrap
- Dinner: Quinoa-Stuffed Bell Peppers
- Snacks: Hummus with Whole Wheat Pita
- Dessert: Mixed Berry Sorbet

Week 4:

Day 22:

- Breakfast: Breakfast Burrito
- Lunch: Quinoa and Black Bean Bowl
- Dinner: Beef and Vegetable Stir-Fry
- Snacks: Cucumber Slices with Tzatziki
- Dessert: Greek Yogurt Cheesecake

Day 23:

- Breakfast: Smoothie Bowl
- Lunch: Caprese Salad
- Dinner: Lemon-Dill Salmon
- Snacks: Cheese and Whole Wheat Crackers
- Dessert: Chia Seed Chocolate Pudding

Day 24:

- Breakfast: Chia Seed Pudding
- Lunch: Tofu Stir-Fry
- Dinner: Spinach and Mushroom Stuffed Chicken
- Snacks: Edamame
- Dessert: Almond Flour Brownies

Day 25:

- Breakfast: Whole Wheat Pancakes
- Lunch: Pork Tenderloin with Roasted Veggies
- Dinner: Cilantro-Lime Black Bean Salad
- Snacks: Mixed Nuts
- Dessert: Banana Nut Muffins

Day 26:

- Breakfast: Breakfast Casserole
- Lunch: Spaghetti Squash with Turkey Meatballs
- Dinner: Roasted Garlic and Rosemary Chicken
- Snacks: Sliced Bell Peppers with Salsa
- Dessert: Oatmeal Raisin Cookies

Day 27:

- Breakfast: Nut Butter and Banana Toast
- Lunch: Baked Eggplant Parmesan
- Dinner: Sweet Potato and Chickpea Tagine
- Snacks: Avocado Salsa
- Dessert: Avocado Chocolate Mousse

Day 28:

- Breakfast: Berry Protein Smoothie
- Lunch: Thai Red Curry with Tofu
- Dinner: Chicken and Veggie Skewers
- Snacks: Baked Sweet Potato Fries
- Dessert: Pumpkin Pie Chia Pudding

Day 29:

- Breakfast: Scrambled Tofu
- Lunch: Tuna Salad Lettuce Wraps
- Dinner: Greek Quinoa Salad
- Snacks: Stuffed Mushrooms
- Dessert: Peach Cobbler

Day 30

- Breakfast: Quinoa and Fruit Bowl
- Lunch: Lentil and Vegetable Soup
- Dinner: Baked Herb-Crusted Cod
- Snacks: Roasted Almonds
- Dessert: Dark Chocolate-Dipped Strawberries

Congratulations on completing the 30-day meal plan! You've enjoyed a wide variety of delicious and diabetes-friendly kidney meals. Remember to adjust portion sizes and ingredients as needed to meet your specific dietary requirements and continue to prioritize your health and well-being.

Chapter 2: Breakfast Recipes

In this chapter, we present a collection of delicious and diabetes-friendly breakfast recipes to kickstart your morning. These recipes are thoughtfully crafted to help you maintain your health while satisfying your taste buds. Let's dive into these flavorful breakfast options.

Vegetable Omelette

Ingredients:

- 2 eggs
- 1/4 cup diced bell peppers
- 1/4 cup diced onions
- 1/4 cup diced tomatoes
- Salt and pepper to taste
- 1 teaspoon olive oil

Instructions:

1. Heat olive oil in a non-stick skillet.
2. Sauté the onions, bell peppers, and tomatoes until tender.

3. Beat the eggs, season with salt and pepper, and pour over the sautéed vegetables.

4. Cook until the omelette is set, then fold it in half and serve.

Cinnamon Oatmeal

Ingredients:

- 1/2 cup old-fashioned oats
- 1 cup water or low-fat milk
- 1/2 teaspoon cinnamon
- 1 tablespoon chopped nuts (optional)
- 1/2 tablespoon honey or a sugar substitute (optional)

Instructions:

1. In a saucepan, bring water or milk to a boil.
2. Stir in oats and reduce heat to low.
3. Cook, stirring occasionally, for about 5 minutes.
4. Add cinnamon and continue cooking until desired consistency.
5. Top with chopped nuts and a drizzle of honey or a sugar substitute.

Greek Yogurt Parfait

Ingredients:

- 1/2 cup Greek yogurt
- 1/4 cup granola (choose a low-sugar variety)
- 1/2 cup mixed berries
- 1 teaspoon honey (optional)

Instructions:

1. In a glass or bowl, layer Greek yogurt, granola, and mixed berries.
2. Drizzle honey on top for a touch of sweetness.

Spinach and Mushroom Frittata

Ingredients:

- 4 eggs
- 1 cup fresh spinach leaves
- 1/2 cup sliced mushrooms
- 1/4 cup diced onions
- Salt and pepper to taste
- 1 teaspoon olive oil

Instructions:

1. Preheat your oven's broiler.
2. In an oven-safe skillet, sauté the onions and mushrooms in olive oil until tender.
3. Add spinach and cook until wilted.
4. Beat the eggs, season with salt and pepper, and pour over the veggies.
5. Cook on the stovetop for a few minutes, then transfer the skillet to the oven.
6. Broil until the frittata is golden and set.

Avocado Toast

Ingredients:

- 1 slice whole wheat bread
- 1/2 ripe avocado
- Salt and pepper to taste
- A pinch of red pepper flakes (optional)
- A drizzle of olive oil

Instructions:

1. Toast the whole wheat bread until golden.
2. Mash the ripe avocado and spread it over the toast.

3. Season with salt, pepper, and red pepper flakes.

4. Drizzle with a touch of olive oil.

Blueberry Quinoa Porridge

Ingredients:

- 1/2 cup cooked quinoa
- 1/2 cup blueberries
- 1/4 cup low-fat milk
- 1 tablespoon honey or a sugar substitute
- A sprinkle of cinnamon

Instructions:

1. In a bowl, combine cooked quinoa and blueberries.

2. Warm the milk and pour it over the quinoa.

3. Sweeten with honey or a sugar substitute and sprinkle with cinnamon.

Breakfast Burrito

Ingredients:

- 2 large eggs
- 1 whole wheat tortilla

- 1/4 cup black beans
- 1/4 cup diced tomatoes
- 1/4 cup diced bell peppers
- 1/4 cup diced onions
- Salt and pepper to taste

Instructions:

1. Scramble the eggs in a pan until cooked.
2. Warm the tortilla in a dry skillet.
3. Fill the tortilla with scrambled eggs, black beans, tomatoes, bell peppers, and onions.
4. Season with salt and pepper, then fold into a burrito.

Smoothie Bowl

Ingredients:

- 1 cup unsweetened almond milk
- 1/2 cup frozen mixed berries
- 1 small banana
- 1 tablespoon chia seeds
- 1 tablespoon almond butter
- 1/4 cup granola (choose a low-sugar variety)

Instructions:

1. Blend almond milk, frozen berries, banana, chia seeds, and almond butter until smooth.

2. Pour the smoothie into a bowl and top with granola.

Chia Seed Pudding

Ingredients:

- 2 tablespoons chia seeds
- 1/2 cup unsweetened almond milk
- 1/2 teaspoon vanilla extract
- 1/2 tablespoon honey or a sugar substitute
- Fresh berries for topping

Instructions:

1. In a jar, combine chia seeds, almond milk, vanilla extract, and sweetener.

2. Stir well and refrigerate overnight.

3. Top with fresh berries before serving.

Whole Wheat Pancakes

Ingredients:

- 1/2 cup whole wheat flour
- 1/2 teaspoon baking powder
- 1/4 teaspoon salt
- 1/2 cup low-fat milk
- 1 egg
- 1/2 tablespoon honey or a sugar substitute
- A touch of vanilla extract

Instructions:

1. In a bowl, whisk together whole wheat flour, baking powder, and salt.
2. In another bowl, mix milk, egg, honey (or sugar substitute), and vanilla extract.
3. Combine wet and dry ingredients and stir until smooth.
4. Cook pancakes on a non-stick skillet until golden.

Breakfast Casserole

Ingredients:

- 4 large eggs
- 1 cup chopped spinach
- 1/2 cup diced bell peppers
- 1/2 cup diced onions
- 1/2 cup low-fat cheese
- Salt and pepper to taste

Instructions:

1. Preheat your oven to 350°F (175°C).
2. In a bowl, beat the eggs and add salt and pepper.
3. Layer a baking dish with spinach, bell peppers, onions, and low-fat cheese.
4. Pour the beaten eggs over the ingredients.
5. Bake for 25-30 minutes until the casserole is set and golden.

Berry Protein Smoothie

Ingredients:

- 1 cup unsweetened almond milk

- 1/2 cup mixed berries
- 1 scoop of protein powder (low sugar)
- 1/2 tablespoon honey or a sugar substitute

Instructions:

1. Blend almond milk, mixed berries, protein powder, and sweetener until smooth.
2. Adjust the sweetness to your preference.

Scrambled Tofu

Ingredients:

- 1/2 block of firm tofu, crumbled
- 1/4 cup diced bell peppers
- 1/4 cup diced onions
- 1/4 cup diced tomatoes
- Turmeric, paprika, salt, and pepper to taste

Instructions:

1. Sauté bell peppers, onions, and tomatoes in a skillet.
2. Add crumbled tofu and season with turmeric, paprika, salt, and pepper.
3. Cook until heated through.

Nut Butter and Banana Toast

Ingredients:

- 1 slice whole wheat bread
- 1 tablespoon nut butter (almond, peanut, etc.)
- 1/2 ripe banana, sliced
- A drizzle of honey or a sugar substitute

Instructions:

1. Toast the whole wheat bread until golden.
2. Spread nut butter over the toast.
3. Top with banana slices and drizzle with honey or a sugar substitute.

Veggie Breakfast Wrap

Ingredients:

- 1 whole wheat tortilla
- 2 large eggs, scrambled
- 1/4 cup diced tomatoes
- 1/4 cup diced bell peppers
- 1/4 cup diced onions
- Salt and pepper to taste

Instructions:

1. Place scrambled eggs on the tortilla.

2. Add diced tomatoes, bell peppers, and onions.

3. Season with salt and pepper.

4. Fold into a wrap.

Sweet Potato Hash

Ingredients:

- 1 medium sweet potato, diced

- 1/4 cup diced onions

- 1/4 cup diced bell peppers

- 1/4 cup black beans (canned and rinsed)

- 1/2 teaspoon paprika

- Salt and pepper to taste

Instructions:

1. Heat a skillet and add a touch of oil.

2. Sauté sweet potatoes, onions, and bell peppers until they begin to soften.

3. Add black beans, paprika, salt, and pepper.

4. Cook until sweet potatoes are tender and slightly crispy.

Egg and Spinach Breakfast Quesadilla

Ingredients:

- 2 whole eggs, scrambled
- 1 whole wheat tortilla
- 1/2 cup fresh spinach leaves
- 1/4 cup low-fat cheese
- Salt and pepper to taste

Instructions:

1. In a skillet, scramble the eggs until cooked.
2. Place the whole wheat tortilla in the skillet and sprinkle one half with cheese.
3. Layer eggs, fresh spinach, and more cheese.
4. Fold the tortilla in half and cook until the cheese melts.

Quinoa and Fruit Bowl

Ingredients:

- 1/2 cup cooked quinoa

- 1/2 cup mixed fresh fruit (e.g., berries, mango, banana)
- 1 tablespoon honey or a sugar substitute
- A sprinkle of cinnamon

Instructions:

1. In a bowl, combine cooked quinoa and mixed fresh fruit.
2. Sweeten with honey or a sugar substitute and sprinkle with cinnamon.
3. Toss to mix and enjoy the refreshing flavors.

Chapter 3: Lunch Recipes

In Chapter 3, we dive into a world of delicious and nutritious lunch options designed with diabetes and kidney health in mind. These recipes are carefully crafted to provide a balance of flavors, textures, and wholesome ingredients. You'll discover a variety of lunch ideas to keep your taste buds excited while maintaining your health.

Grilled Chicken Salad

Ingredients:

- 2 boneless, skinless chicken breasts
- 1 tablespoon olive oil
- Salt and pepper to taste
- 4 cups mixed greens
- 1 cup cherry tomatoes, halved
- 1/2 cucumber, sliced
- 1/4 red onion, thinly sliced
- 2 tablespoons balsamic vinaigrette

Instructions:

1. Preheat your grill to medium-high heat.
2. Brush chicken breasts with olive oil and season with salt and pepper.
3. Grill the chicken for about 6-7 minutes per side or until fully cooked.
4. Let the chicken rest for a few minutes, then slice it.
5. In a large bowl, combine mixed greens, cherry tomatoes, cucumber, and red onion.
6. Top with grilled chicken slices and drizzle with balsamic vinaigrette.

Lentil and Vegetable Soup

Ingredients:

- 1 cup dried green lentils
- 6 cups vegetable broth
- 1 onion, chopped
- 2 carrots, sliced
- 2 celery stalks, chopped
- 1 can diced tomatoes
- 2 cloves garlic, minced
- 1 teaspoon cumin

- 1/2 teaspoon paprika
- Salt and pepper to taste
- Fresh parsley for garnish

Instructions:

1. In a large pot, sauté the onion, carrots, and celery until softened.
2. Add garlic, cumin, and paprika. Cook for another minute.
3. Rinse lentils and add them to the pot.
4. Pour in vegetable broth and diced tomatoes.
5. Bring to a boil, then reduce heat and simmer for about 30 minutes.
6. Season with salt and pepper, and garnish with fresh parsley.

Turkey and Avocado Wrap

Ingredients:

- 4 whole-grain tortillas
- 1 cup sliced turkey breast
- 1 avocado, sliced
- 1 cup mixed greens

- 1/4 cup plain Greek yogurt

- 1 teaspoon Dijon mustard

- Salt and pepper to taste

Instructions:

1. In a small bowl, mix Greek yogurt, Dijon mustard, salt, and pepper to make a dressing.

2. Lay out the tortillas and divide turkey, avocado, and mixed greens among them.

3. Drizzle the dressing over the fillings.

4. Fold the sides of the tortillas and roll them up.

Quinoa and Black Bean Bowl

Ingredients:

- 1 cup quinoa

- 2 cups water

- 1 can black beans, drained and rinsed

- 1 cup corn kernels (frozen or canned)

- 1 red bell pepper, diced

- 1/4 cup fresh cilantro, chopped

- Juice of 1 lime

- 1 tablespoon olive oil

- Salt and pepper to taste

Instructions:

1. Rinse quinoa under cold water and combine it with 2 cups of water in a saucepan.
2. Bring to a boil, then reduce heat, cover, and simmer for 15 minutes.
3. In a large bowl, combine cooked quinoa, black beans, corn, and red bell pepper.
4. In a separate small bowl, whisk together lime juice, olive oil, salt, and pepper.
5. Pour the dressing over the quinoa mixture, add cilantro, and toss to combine.

Salmon with Asparagus

Ingredients:

- 2 salmon fillets
- 1 bunch asparagus, trimmed
- 2 tablespoons olive oil
- 2 cloves garlic, minced
- 1 lemon, sliced
- Salt and pepper to taste

Instructions:

1. Preheat your oven to 400°F (200°C).
2. Place salmon fillets and asparagus on a baking sheet.
3. Drizzle with olive oil and sprinkle minced garlic, salt, and pepper.
4. Lay lemon slices over the salmon.
5. Bake for about 15-20 minutes or until the salmon flakes easily with a fork.

Tofu Stir-Fry

Ingredients:

-   14 oz (400g) firm tofu, cubed
-   2 cups mixed stir-fry vegetables (broccoli, bell peppers, snap peas, etc.)
-   2 tablespoons low-sodium soy sauce
-   1 tablespoon hoisin sauce
-   1 tablespoon sesame oil
-   1 clove garlic, minced
-   1/2 teaspoon ginger, grated
-   Cooked brown rice or quinoa

Instructions:

1. In a large pan, heat sesame oil over medium-high heat.
2. Add cubed tofu and stir-fry until golden brown.
3. Remove tofu from the pan and set aside.
4. In the same pan, add garlic and ginger, then the mixed vegetables.
5. Stir-fry for a few minutes until the veggies are tender.
6. Return tofu to the pan, add soy sauce and hoisin sauce.
7. Cook for a few more minutes.
8. Serve over cooked brown rice or quinoa.

Caprese Salad

Ingredients:

- 4 ripe tomatoes, sliced
- 8 oz (225g) fresh mozzarella cheese, sliced
- Fresh basil leaves
- 2 tablespoons extra-virgin olive oil
- 1 tablespoon balsamic vinegar
- Salt and pepper to taste

Instructions:

1. Arrange tomato and mozzarella slices on a serving plate.
2. Tuck fresh basil leaves between the slices.
3. Drizzle with olive oil and balsamic vinegar.
4. Season with salt and pepper to taste.

Minestrone Soup

Ingredients:

- 1 tablespoon olive oil
- 1 onion, chopped
- 2 carrots, sliced
- 2 celery stalks, chopped
- 2 cloves garlic, minced
- 1 can kidney beans, drained and rinsed
- 1 can diced tomatoes
- 4 cups vegetable broth
- 1 cup small pasta (e.g., ditalini)
- 2 cups spinach
- 1/4 cup grated Parmesan cheese
- Salt and pepper to taste

Instructions:

1. In a large pot, heat olive oil over medium heat.
2. Add onion, carrots, and celery. Sauté until softened.
3. Add garlic and cook for another minute.
4. Stir in kidney beans, diced tomatoes, vegetable broth, and pasta.
5. Simmer for about 10-15 minutes or until the pasta is tender.
6. Add spinach and cook until wilted.
7. Serve hot with a sprinkle of grated Parmesan cheese.

Chickpea and Spinach Salad

Ingredients:

- 1 can chickpeas, drained and rinsed
- 2 cups fresh spinach
- 1/2 red onion, finely chopped
- 1 cucumber, diced
- 1/4 cup feta cheese, crumbled
- 2 tablespoons balsamic vinaigrette
- Salt and pepper to taste

Instructions:

1. In a large salad bowl, combine chickpeas, fresh spinach, red onion, and cucumber.
2. Sprinkle with feta cheese.
3. Drizzle with balsamic vinaigrette.
4. Season with salt and pepper to taste.

Veggie and Hummus Wrap

Ingredients:

- 4 whole-grain tortillas
- 1 cup hummus
- 2 cups mixed salad greens
- 1 bell pepper, sliced
- 1 cucumber, sliced
- 1/2 cup shredded carrots
- Salt and pepper to taste

Instructions:

1. Spread a generous layer of hummus on each tortilla.
2. Lay out mixed salad greens, bell pepper, cucumber, and shredded carrots.
3. Season with salt and pepper to taste.

4. Roll up the tortillas and enjoy!

Teriyaki Chicken Bowl

Ingredients:

- 2 boneless, skinless chicken breasts
- 1 cup broccoli florets
- 1 cup snap peas
- 1 cup brown rice
- 2 tablespoons low-sodium teriyaki sauce

Instructions:

1. Cook brown rice according to package instructions.
2. In a non-stick pan, cook chicken until no longer pink.
3. Add broccoli and snap peas and stir-fry for a few minutes.
4. Pour teriyaki sauce over the chicken and vegetables.
5. Serve the teriyaki chicken over cooked brown rice.

Zucchini Noodles with Pesto

Ingredients:

- 2 large zucchinis, spiralized into noodles

- 1/2 cup cherry tomatoes, halved
- 1/4 cup pine nuts
- 1/4 cup basil pesto
- Grated Parmesan cheese for garnish
- Salt and pepper to taste

Instructions:

1. In a pan, lightly sauté zucchini noodles for a few minutes.
2. Toss in cherry tomatoes and pine nuts.
3. Stir in basil pesto.
4. Season with salt and pepper.
5. Serve with a sprinkle of grated Parmesan cheese.

Turkey and Cranberry Quinoa Salad

Ingredients:

- 2 cups cooked quinoa
- 1 cup cooked turkey, diced
- 1/2 cup dried cranberries
- 1/4 cup sliced almonds
- 1/4 cup fresh parsley, chopped
- 2 tablespoons balsamic vinaigrette

- Salt and pepper to taste

Instructions:

1. In a large bowl, combine cooked quinoa, diced turkey, dried cranberries, sliced almonds, and fresh parsley.
2. Drizzle with balsamic vinaigrette.
3. Season with salt and pepper to taste.

Tuna Salad Lettuce Wraps

Ingredients:

- 2 cans of tuna, drained
- 1/4 cup plain Greek yogurt
- 1/4 cup diced celery
- 1/4 cup diced red onion
- 1 teaspoon Dijon mustard
- Lettuce leaves for wrapping

Instructions:

1. In a bowl, mix tuna, Greek yogurt, diced celery, red onion, and Dijon mustard.

2. Spoon the tuna salad into lettuce leaves and wrap them up for a low-carb lunch.

Spicy Cauliflower Soup

Ingredients:

- 1 head of cauliflower, chopped
- 1 onion, chopped
- 2 cloves garlic, minced
- 4 cups vegetable broth
- 1/2 teaspoon curry powder
- 1/4 teaspoon cayenne pepper
- Salt and pepper to taste

Instructions:

1. In a large pot, sauté onion and garlic until soft.
2. Add chopped cauliflower, vegetable broth, curry powder, and cayenne pepper.
3. Bring to a boil, then reduce heat and simmer for about 20 minutes.
4. Use a blender to puree the soup until smooth.
5. Season with salt and pepper.

Shrimp and Broccoli Stir-Fry

Ingredients:

- 8 oz (225g) shrimp, peeled and deveined
- 2 cups broccoli florets
- 1 red bell pepper, sliced
- 2 tablespoons low-sodium soy sauce
- 1 tablespoon honey
- 1 clove garlic, minced
- 1/2 teaspoon ginger, grated
- Cooked brown rice

Instructions:

1. In a large pan, heat olive oil over medium-high heat.
2. Stir-fry shrimp, broccoli, and red bell pepper until shrimp turn pink and veggies are tender.
3. In a small bowl, mix soy sauce, honey, garlic, and ginger.
4. Pour the sauce over the stir-fry.
5. Serve over cooked brown rice.

Greek Quinoa Salad

Ingredients:

- 1 cup cooked quinoa
- 1 cup cucumber, diced
- 1 cup cherry tomatoes, halved
- 1/2 cup kalamata olives, pitted and sliced
- 1/4 cup red onion, finely chopped
- 1/4 cup feta cheese, crumbled
- 2 tablespoons olive oil
- Juice of 1 lemon
- 1 teaspoon dried oregano
- Salt and pepper to taste

Instructions:

1. In a large bowl, combine cooked quinoa, diced cucumber, cherry tomatoes, kalamata olives, red onion, and feta cheese.
2. Drizzle with olive oil and lemon juice.
3. Season with dried oregano, salt, and pepper to taste.

Eggplant and Tomato Stack

Ingredients:

- 2 eggplants, sliced into rounds
- 2 large tomatoes, sliced
- 1/2 cup fresh basil leaves
- 1/4 cup grated Parmesan cheese
- 1/4 cup balsamic vinegar
- 2 tablespoons olive oil
- Salt and pepper to taste

Instructions:

1. Preheat your oven to 350°F (175°C).
2. Brush eggplant slices with olive oil and season with salt and pepper.
3. Bake for about 20 minutes until softened.
4. In a baking dish, stack eggplant rounds, tomato slices, and basil leaves.
5. Sprinkle with grated Parmesan cheese.
6. Drizzle with balsamic vinegar.
7. Bake for an additional 10-15 minutes.
8. Serve these flavorful stacks warm.

Chapter 4: Dinner Recipes

In this chapter, you'll discover a selection of delectable dinner recipes that are not only delicious but also diabetes-friendly and gentle on your kidneys. Each recipe is carefully crafted to balance flavors, nutrients, and dietary considerations. So, let's dive into these delightful dinner options that will make your evening meals both satisfying and nutritious.

Baked Herb-Crusted Cod

Ingredients:

- 4 cod fillets
- 1/4 cup breadcrumbs (whole wheat)
- 2 tablespoons fresh parsley, chopped
- 2 tablespoons fresh dill, chopped
- 1 clove garlic, minced
- 1 lemon, zest and juice
- 2 tablespoons olive oil
- Salt and pepper to taste

Instructions:

1. Preheat your oven to 375°F (190°C).

2. In a bowl, combine breadcrumbs, parsley, dill, garlic, lemon zest, and a pinch of salt and pepper.

3. Brush the cod fillets with olive oil, then coat them with the breadcrumb mixture.

4. Place the fillets on a baking sheet and drizzle with lemon juice.

5. Bake for 15-20 minutes or until the cod flakes easily with a fork.

Chicken and Veggie Skewers

Ingredients:

- 2 boneless, skinless chicken breasts, cut into cubes
- 1 red bell pepper, cut into chunks
- 1 green bell pepper, cut into chunks
- 1 red onion, cut into chunks
- 2 zucchinis, sliced
- 2 tablespoons olive oil
- 1 teaspoon dried oregano
- Salt and pepper to taste

Instructions:

1. Preheat your grill to medium-high heat.

2. Thread chicken and vegetables onto skewers.

3. In a small bowl, mix olive oil, oregano, salt, and pepper.

4. Brush the skewers with the olive oil mixture.

5. Grill for 10-15 minutes, turning occasionally, until the chicken is cooked through and the vegetables are tender.

Quinoa-Stuffed Bell Peppers

Ingredients:

- 4 bell peppers, tops removed and seeds removed
- 1 cup quinoa, cooked
- 1 cup black beans, drained and rinsed
- 1 cup corn (frozen or canned)
- 1 cup diced tomatoes
- 1 teaspoon cumin
- 1/2 teaspoon chili powder
- Salt and pepper to taste
- 1/2 cup shredded low-fat cheddar cheese (optional)

Instructions:

1. Preheat your oven to 375°F (190°C).

2. In a large bowl, combine cooked quinoa, black beans, corn, diced tomatoes, cumin, chili powder, salt, and pepper.

3. Stuff each bell pepper with the quinoa mixture.

4. Place the stuffed peppers in a baking dish, and cover with aluminum foil.

5. Bake for 25-30 minutes, or until the peppers are tender.

6. If desired, top with shredded cheddar cheese and bake for an additional 5 minutes, or until cheese is melted.

Beef and Vegetable Stir-Fry

Ingredients:

- 1 pound lean beef (sirloin or flank steak), thinly sliced
- 2 cups broccoli florets
- 1 red bell pepper, sliced
- 1 yellow bell pepper, sliced
- 1/2 cup low-sodium soy sauce

- 2 tablespoons honey
- 1 tablespoon cornstarch
- 1 tablespoon ginger, minced
- 2 cloves garlic, minced
- 2 tablespoons vegetable oil
- Sesame seeds for garnish (optional)

Instructions:

1. In a small bowl, whisk together soy sauce, honey, cornstarch, ginger, and garlic.
2. Heat vegetable oil in a large skillet or wok over high heat.
3. Add sliced beef and stir-fry until browned.
4. Add the vegetables and continue to stir-fry for a few minutes.
5. Pour the sauce over the beef and vegetables and cook until the sauce thickens.
6. Serve hot, garnished with sesame seeds if desired.

Garlic and Herb Shrimp

Ingredients:

- 1 pound large shrimp, peeled and deveined

- 2 tablespoons olive oil
- 4 cloves garlic, minced
- 1/4 cup fresh parsley, chopped
- 1 lemon, juice and zest
- Salt and pepper to taste

Instructions:

1. In a large skillet, heat olive oil over medium heat.
2. Add minced garlic and sauté until fragrant.
3. Add the shrimp and cook until they turn pink and opaque.
4. Stir in lemon juice, lemon zest, and fresh parsley.
5. Season with salt and pepper to taste.
6. Serve hot with your choice of side vegetables or grains.

Spinach and Mushroom Stuffed Chicken

Ingredients:

- 4 boneless, skinless chicken breasts
- 2 cups fresh spinach, chopped

- 1 cup mushrooms, sliced
- 1/4 cup low-fat cream cheese
- 2 cloves garlic, minced
- Salt and pepper to taste
- Toothpicks or kitchen twine

Instructions:

1. Preheat your oven to 375°F (190°C).
2. In a skillet, sauté mushrooms and garlic until they're tender and moisture has evaporated.
3. Stir in chopped spinach and cook for a few more minutes until wilted.
4. Season with salt and pepper.
5. Butterfly each chicken breast and spread a layer of cream cheese on the inside.
6. Spoon the mushroom and spinach mixture onto each chicken breast and fold them closed.
7. Secure with toothpicks or kitchen twine.
8. Bake for 25-30 minutes or until the chicken is cooked through.

Lemon-Dill Salmon

Ingredients:

- 4 salmon fillets
- 2 tablespoons olive oil
- 2 tablespoons fresh dill, chopped
- 1 lemon, zest and juice
- Salt and pepper to taste

Instructions:

1. Preheat your oven to 375°F (190°C).
2. Place the salmon fillets on a baking sheet.
3. Drizzle with olive oil, then sprinkle with dill, lemon zest, lemon juice, salt, and pepper.
4. Bake for 15-20 minutes or until the salmon flakes easily with a fork.

Vegetable Curry

Ingredients:

- 2 cups mixed vegetables (e.g., bell peppers, carrots, zucchini)
- 1 onion, chopped

- 2 cloves garlic, minced
- 1 can of chickpeas, drained and rinsed
- 1 can of diced tomatoes
- 1 cup low-sodium vegetable broth
- 2 tablespoons curry powder
- Salt and pepper to taste
- 1 cup cooked brown rice or quinoa (for serving)

Instructions:

1. In a large pot, sauté the onion and garlic until fragrant.
2. Add the mixed vegetables and cook for a few minutes.
3. Stir in the chickpeas, diced tomatoes, vegetable broth, and curry powder.
4. Season with salt and pepper.
5. Simmer for about 20-25 minutes until the vegetables are tender.
6. Serve over cooked brown rice or quinoa.

Mushroom and Lentil Shepherd's Pie

Ingredients:

- 1 cup brown or green lentils, cooked
- 2 cups mushrooms, chopped
- 1 onion, chopped
- 2 cloves garlic, minced
- 1 cup frozen peas and carrots
- 1 cup low-sodium vegetable broth
- 1 teaspoon thyme
- Mashed sweet potatoes (for topping)
- Salt and pepper to taste

Instructions:

1. Preheat your oven to 375°F (190°C).
2. In a skillet, sauté the mushrooms, onion, and garlic until tender.
3. Add the cooked lentils, peas, carrots, vegetable broth, and thyme.
4. Season with salt and pepper.
5. Transfer the mixture to a baking dish and top with mashed sweet potatoes.
6. Bake for 20-25 minutes, or until the top is golden.

Spaghetti Squash with Turkey Meatballs

Ingredients:

- 1 spaghetti squash, halved and seeds removed
- 1 pound lean ground turkey
- 1/4 cup whole wheat breadcrumbs
- 1/4 cup grated Parmesan cheese
- 1 egg
- 1 can of low-sodium tomato sauce
- 1 teaspoon Italian seasoning
- Salt and pepper to taste

Instructions:

1. Preheat your oven to 375°F (190°C).
2. Place the squash halves cut side down on a baking sheet and roast for 30-40 minutes until tender.
3. In a bowl, combine ground turkey, breadcrumbs, Parmesan cheese, egg, Italian seasoning, salt, and pepper.
4. Shape the mixture into meatballs.
5. In a skillet, cook the meatballs until browned, then add tomato sauce and simmer.

6. Serve the meatballs and sauce over cooked spaghetti squash.

Tofu and Vegetable Stir-Fry

Ingredients:

- 14 ounces extra-firm tofu, cubed
- 2 cups broccoli florets
- 1 red bell pepper, sliced
- 1 yellow bell pepper, sliced
- 1 cup snap peas
- 2 tablespoons low-sodium soy sauce
- 1 tablespoon hoisin sauce
- 1 teaspoon ginger, minced
- 1 teaspoon garlic, minced
- 2 tablespoons vegetable oil
- Cooked brown rice or quinoa (for serving)

Instructions:

1. In a large skillet or wok, heat vegetable oil over medium-high heat.
2. Add tofu cubes and stir-fry until they are lightly browned.

3. Add broccoli, bell peppers, and snap peas. Continue stir-frying until vegetables are tender.

4. In a small bowl, mix together soy sauce, hoisin sauce, ginger, and garlic.

5. Pour the sauce over the tofu and vegetables.

6. Serve hot over cooked brown rice or quinoa.

Pork Tenderloin with Roasted Veggies

Ingredients:

- 1 pork tenderloin
- 2 cups mixed vegetables (e.g., carrots, potatoes, Brussels sprouts)
- 2 tablespoons olive oil
- 1 teaspoon rosemary
- 1 teaspoon thyme
- Salt and pepper to taste

Instructions:

1. Preheat your oven to 375°F (190°C).

2. Season the pork tenderloin with rosemary, thyme, salt, and pepper.

3. Place the seasoned pork and mixed vegetables on a baking sheet.

4. Drizzle with olive oil.

5. Roast for 30-35 minutes, or until the pork is cooked and the vegetables are tender.

Cilantro-Lime Black Bean Salad

Ingredients:

- 2 cans of black beans, drained and rinsed
- 1 cup corn (frozen or canned)
- 1 red bell pepper, chopped
- 1/2 red onion, chopped
- 1/4 cup fresh cilantro, chopped
- 2 tablespoons olive oil
- 2 limes, juice and zest
- Salt and pepper to taste

Instructions:

1. In a large bowl, combine black beans, corn, red bell pepper, red onion, and cilantro.

2. In a small bowl, whisk together olive oil, lime juice, lime zest, salt, and pepper.

3. Pour the dressing over the salad and toss to combine.

4. Chill in the refrigerator for a while before serving.

Roasted Garlic and Rosemary Chicken

Ingredients:

- 4 chicken breasts
- 1 head of garlic, cloves separated and peeled
- 2 tablespoons olive oil
- 2 sprigs fresh rosemary
- Salt and pepper to taste

Instructions:

1. Preheat your oven to 375°F (190°C).

2. Place the chicken breasts on a baking sheet.

3. Tuck garlic cloves and rosemary sprigs under and around the chicken.

4. Drizzle with olive oil and season with salt and pepper.

5. Roast for 30-35 minutes or until the chicken is cooked through.

Teriyaki Portobello Mushrooms

Ingredients:

- 4 large portobello mushrooms
- 1/4 cup low-sodium teriyaki sauce
- 2 tablespoons olive oil
- 1 tablespoon sesame seeds
- Salt and pepper to taste

Instructions:

1. Preheat your grill or broiler.
2. Clean the portobello mushrooms and remove the stems.
3. In a small bowl, mix teriyaki sauce, olive oil, sesame seeds, salt, and pepper.
4. Brush the mushroom caps with the teriyaki mixture.
5. Grill or broil the mushrooms for 4-5 minutes on each side or until tender.

Baked Eggplant Parmesan

Ingredients:

- 2 large eggplants, sliced
- 2 cups whole wheat breadcrumbs
- 2 cups marinara sauce (low-sodium)
- 1 cup shredded mozzarella cheese (part-skim)
- 1/2 cup grated Parmesan cheese
- 1 teaspoon dried basil
- 1 teaspoon dried oregano
- Salt and pepper to taste

Instructions:

1. Preheat your oven to 375°F (190°C).
2. Dip eggplant slices in breadcrumbs and arrange them on a baking sheet.
3. Bake for 20 minutes, flipping once, until they are golden.
4. In a baking dish, layer eggplant slices, marinara sauce, mozzarella, Parmesan, basil, oregano, salt, and pepper.
5. Repeat the layers.

6. Bake for 25-30 minutes or until the cheese is melted and bubbly.

Thai Red Curry with Tofu

Ingredients:

- 1 package extra-firm tofu, cubed
- 1 can of coconut milk
- 2 tablespoons red curry paste
- 1 red bell pepper, sliced
- 1 zucchini, sliced
- 1 cup snow peas
- 1 tablespoon fish sauce (or soy sauce for a vegetarian option)
- 1 tablespoon brown sugar
- 1 lime, juice and zest
- Fresh cilantro (for garnish)
- Cooked brown rice (for serving)

Instructions:

1. In a large skillet, heat the coconut milk and red curry paste.
2. Add tofu, red bell pepper, zucchini, and snow peas.

3. Simmer until the vegetables are tender.

4. Stir in fish sauce, brown sugar, lime juice, and lime zest.

5. Serve the curry over cooked brown rice, garnished with fresh cilantro.

Sweet Potato and Chickpea Tagine

Ingredients:

- 2 sweet potatoes, peeled and diced
- 1 can of chickpeas, drained and rinsed
- 1 onion, chopped
- 2 cloves garlic, minced
- 1 can of diced tomatoes
- 2 teaspoons ground cumin
- 1 teaspoon ground cinnamon
- Salt and pepper to taste
- Fresh cilantro (for garnish)
- Cooked couscous or quinoa (for serving)

Instructions:

1. In a large pot, sauté the onion and garlic until fragrant.

2. Add sweet potatoes, chickpeas, diced tomatoes, cumin, cinnamon, salt, and pepper.

3. Simmer until the sweet potatoes are tender.

4. Serve over cooked couscous or quinoa, garnished with fresh cilantro.

Chapter 5: Snacks and Appetizers

In this chapter, we've curated a collection of snacks and appetizers that are perfect for satisfying those cravings without compromising your health. These options are packed with flavor, easy to prepare, and designed to keep your blood sugar levels in check.

Roasted Almonds

Ingredients:

- 1 cup raw almonds
- 1 tablespoon olive oil
- 1/2 teaspoon sea salt

Instructions:

1. Preheat your oven to 350°F (175°C).
2. In a bowl, toss the almonds with olive oil and sea salt.
3. Spread them on a baking sheet and roast for about 15 minutes or until fragrant and slightly browned. Let them cool before serving.

Guacamole and Veggie Sticks

Ingredients:

- 2 ripe avocados
- 1 small tomato, diced
- 1/4 cup finely chopped red onion
- 1 clove garlic, minced
- Juice of 1 lime
- Salt and pepper to taste
- Carrot, cucumber, and bell pepper sticks for dipping

Instructions:

1. Mash the avocados in a bowl.
2. Add the diced tomato, red onion, minced garlic, and lime juice. Mix well.
3. Season with salt and pepper to taste.
4. Serve with a colorful array of carrot, cucumber, and bell pepper sticks.

Hummus with Whole Wheat Pita

Ingredients:

- 1 cup canned chickpeas, drained and rinsed

- 2 tablespoons tahini
- 2 cloves garlic, minced
- 2 tablespoons lemon juice
- 2 tablespoons olive oil
- 1/2 teaspoon ground cumin
- Salt to taste
- Whole wheat pita bread, cut into triangles for dipping

Instructions:

1. In a food processor, combine the chickpeas, tahini, minced garlic, lemon juice, olive oil, ground cumin, and a pinch of salt.
2. Blend until smooth and creamy.
3. Serve with whole wheat pita triangles.

Cucumber Slices with Tzatziki

Ingredients:

- 1 cucumber, thinly sliced
- 1 cup Greek yogurt
- 2 cloves garlic, minced
- 1 tablespoon fresh dill, chopped
- 1 tablespoon lemon juice

- Salt and pepper to taste

Instructions:

1. In a bowl, combine Greek yogurt, minced garlic, fresh dill, lemon juice, salt, and pepper.
2. Stir until well mixed.
3. Serve the sliced cucumber with the tzatziki sauce.

Deviled Eggs

Ingredients:

- 6 hard-boiled eggs
- 2 tablespoons mayonnaise
- 1 teaspoon Dijon mustard
- 1/2 teaspoon paprika
- Salt and pepper to taste
- Chopped chives for garnish

Instructions:

1. Cut the hard-boiled eggs in half and remove the yolks.
2. Mash the yolks and combine them with mayonnaise, Dijon mustard, paprika, salt, and pepper.

3. Fill the egg whites with the yolk mixture and garnish
    with chopped chives.

Edamame

Ingredients:

- 1 cup frozen edamame
- 1 tablespoon olive oil
- Sea salt

Instructions:

1. Cook the edamame according to package
    instructions.
2. Toss the cooked edamame in olive oil and sprinkle
    with sea salt.

Cheese and Whole Wheat Crackers

Ingredients:

- Assorted low-fat cheeses
- Whole wheat crackers

Instructions:

1. Arrange an assortment of low-fat cheeses on a platter.
2. Serve with whole wheat crackers.

Greek Yogurt with Berries

Ingredients:

- 1 cup Greek yogurt
- Fresh mixed berries (strawberries, blueberries, raspberries)
- Honey for drizzling (optional)

Instructions:

1. Spoon Greek yogurt into a bowl.
2. Top with fresh mixed berries.
3. Drizzle with honey if desired.

Mixed Nuts

Ingredients:

- A mixture of unsalted nuts (almonds, walnuts, cashews)

Instructions:

1. Create your own mix of unsalted nuts.
2. Portion them into small, snack-sized bags for easy and healthy snacking.

Sliced Bell Peppers with Salsa

Ingredients:

*   Red, yellow, and green bell peppers, sliced
*   Fresh salsa for dipping

Instructions:

1. Slice the bell peppers into strips.
2. Serve with fresh salsa for dipping.

Avocado Salsa

Ingredients:

*   2 ripe avocados, diced
*   1/2 red onion, finely chopped
*   1 tomato, diced
*   1/4 cup cilantro, chopped
*   Juice of 1 lime

- Salt and pepper to taste

Instructions:

1. In a bowl, gently mix the diced avocados, chopped red onion, diced tomato, cilantro, lime juice, salt, and pepper.
2. Serve with whole grain tortilla chips.

Caprese Skewers

Ingredients:

- Cherry tomatoes
- Fresh mozzarella balls
- Fresh basil leaves
- Balsamic glaze for drizzling

Instructions:

1. Thread a cherry tomato, a mozzarella ball, and a fresh basil leaf onto a skewer.
2. Drizzle with balsamic glaze.

Baked Sweet Potato Fries

Ingredients:

- Sweet potatoes, cut into fries
- Olive oil
- Paprika
- Salt and pepper to taste

Instructions:

1. Preheat your oven to 425°F (220°C).
2. Toss the sweet potato fries with olive oil, paprika, salt, and pepper.
3. Bake until crispy, about 30 minutes.

Spinach and Artichoke Dip

Ingredients:

- 1 cup spinach, cooked and chopped
- 1/2 cup canned artichoke hearts, drained and chopped
- 1 cup Greek yogurt
- 1/2 cup light cream cheese
- 1/4 cup grated Parmesan cheese

- 2 cloves garlic, minced

Instructions:

1. Mix the cooked and chopped spinach, chopped artichoke hearts, Greek yogurt, light cream cheese, grated Parmesan cheese, and minced garlic in a bowl.

2. Heat in the oven until bubbly and serve with vegetable sticks or whole wheat pita.

Stuffed Mushrooms

Ingredients:

- Large mushrooms, stems removed
- Cream cheese
- Minced garlic
- Chopped fresh herbs (e.g., parsley or chives)

Instructions:

1. Mix cream cheese, minced garlic, and chopped herbs.

2. Stuff the mushroom caps with the cream cheese mixture.

3. Bake until mushrooms are tender.

Quinoa Salad Cups

Ingredients:

- Cooked quinoa
- Chopped fresh vegetables (e.g., cucumber, cherry tomatoes, bell peppers)
- Balsamic vinaigrette

Instructions:

1. Fill small cups or lettuce leaves with cooked quinoa and chopped fresh vegetables.
2. Drizzle with balsamic vinaigrette.

Chicken Lettuce Wraps

Ingredients:

- Ground chicken
- Diced water chestnuts
- Soy sauce
- Hoisin sauce
- Sesame oil
- Lettuce leaves for wrapping

Instructions:

1. Cook ground chicken with diced water chestnuts, soy sauce, hoisin sauce, and sesame oil.

2. Spoon the mixture into lettuce leaves and wrap.

Cottage Cheese with Pineapple

Ingredients:

- Low-fat cottage cheese
- Fresh pineapple chunks

Instructions:

1. Serve low-fat cottage cheese with fresh pineapple chunks.

Chapter 6: Desserts

Indulging your sweet tooth while maintaining a diabetes-friendly diet has never been this delightful. These dessert recipes are designed to satisfy your cravings without spiking your blood sugar. From fruity parfaits to rich chocolate treats, you'll find a variety of options to choose from. Let's dive into these delectable desserts.

Berry Parfait

Ingredients:

- 1 cup of mixed berries (strawberries, blueberries, raspberries)
- 1 cup of Greek yogurt
- 2 tablespoons of crushed almonds
- 1 teaspoon of honey (optional)

Instructions:

1. In a glass or bowl, layer Greek yogurt at the bottom.
2. Add a layer of mixed berries.
3. Repeat the layers.

4. Top with crushed almonds and a drizzle of honey (if desired).

5. Serve chilled.

Dark Chocolate-Dipped Strawberries

Ingredients:

- 12 fresh strawberries
- 3 ounces of dark chocolate (70% cocoa or higher)

Instructions:

1. Melt the dark chocolate in a microwave-safe bowl in 20-second intervals, stirring until smooth.

2. Dip each strawberry into the melted chocolate, covering half of the strawberry.

3. Place them on a parchment-lined tray.

4. Let them cool and harden in the refrigerator.

5. Enjoy this guilt-free chocolate treat.

Baked Apples with Cinnamon

Ingredients:

- 2 apples (your choice of variety)

- 1 teaspoon of ground cinnamon
- 1 tablespoon of chopped walnuts (optional)

Instructions:

1. Preheat your oven to 350°F (175°C).
2. Core the apples and place them in an oven-safe dish.
3. Sprinkle with ground cinnamon and add chopped walnuts if desired.
4. Bake for about 20-25 minutes or until apples are soft.
5. Serve warm.

Greek Yogurt Cheesecake

Ingredients:

- 1 cup of Greek yogurt
- 1/4 cup of cream cheese
- 2 tablespoons of honey
- 1 teaspoon of vanilla extract

Instructions:

1. In a bowl, combine Greek yogurt, cream cheese, honey, and vanilla extract.
2. Mix until smooth.

3. Pour the mixture into small serving cups or bowls.

4. Refrigerate for a few hours until set.

5. Top with fresh berries or a drizzle of honey if desired.

Sugar-Free Pudding

Ingredients:

- 1 cup of unsweetened almond milk
- 2 tablespoons of unsweetened cocoa powder
- 2 tablespoons of cornstarch
- 1/4 cup of sweetener (stevia or erythritol)
- 1 teaspoon of vanilla extract

Instructions:

1. In a saucepan, whisk together almond milk, cocoa powder, cornstarch, and sweetener.

2. Heat over medium heat, stirring constantly until the mixture thickens.

3. Remove from heat, add vanilla extract, and stir.

4. Pour into serving cups and refrigerate until set.

Almond Flour Brownies

Ingredients:

- 1 cup of almond flour
- 1/4 cup of unsweetened cocoa powder
- 1/2 cup of sweetener (stevia or erythritol)
- 1/4 cup of melted coconut oil
- 2 large eggs
- 1 teaspoon of vanilla extract

Instructions:

1. Preheat your oven to 350°F (175°C) and grease a baking dish.
2. In a bowl, combine almond flour, cocoa powder, sweetener, coconut oil, eggs, and vanilla extract.
3. Mix until well combined.
4. Pour the batter into the baking dish.
5. Bake for 20-25 minutes or until a toothpick comes out clean.
6. Allow to cool before cutting into brownie squares.

Chia Seed Chocolate Pudding

Ingredients:

- 2 tablespoons of chia seeds
- 1 cup of unsweetened almond milk
- 2 tablespoons of unsweetened cocoa powder
- 1/4 cup of sweetener (stevia or erythritol)
- 1/2 teaspoon of vanilla extract

Instructions:

1. In a jar, combine chia seeds, almond milk, cocoa powder, sweetener, and vanilla extract.
2. Stir well.
3. Refrigerate overnight or for at least 2 hours until the pudding thickens.
4. Top with berries or nuts before serving.

Mixed Berry Sorbet

Ingredients:

- 2 cups of mixed berries (strawberries, blueberries, raspberries)
- 1/4 cup of sweetener (stevia or erythritol)

- 1 tablespoon of lemon juice

Instructions:

1. Place the mixed berries, sweetener, and lemon juice
    in a blender.
2. Blend until smooth.
3. Pour the mixture into a shallow container and freeze
    for a few hours, stirring occasionally.
4. Scoop and serve.

Banana Nut Muffins

Ingredients:

- 2 ripe bananas, mashed
- 2 eggs
- 1/4 cup almond flour
- 1/4 cup coconut flour
- 1/4 cup chopped walnuts
- 1 teaspoon baking soda
- 1/2 teaspoon cinnamon
- 1/4 cup sweetener (stevia or erythritol)
- 1 teaspoon vanilla extract

Instructions:

1. Preheat your oven to 350°F (175°C) and line a muffin tin with paper liners.
2. In a bowl, combine mashed bananas, eggs, almond flour, coconut flour, chopped walnuts, baking soda, cinnamon, sweetener, and vanilla extract.
3. Mix until well combined.
4. Divide the batter into the muffin cups.
5. Bake for 20-25 minutes or until a toothpick comes out clean.
6. Let them cool before enjoying.

Oatmeal Raisin Cookies

Ingredients:

- 1 cup rolled oats
- 1/4 cup almond flour
- 1/4 cup raisins
- 1/4 cup unsweetened applesauce
- 1/4 cup sweetener (stevia or erythritol)
- 1/2 teaspoon cinnamon
- 1/2 teaspoon vanilla extract

Instructions:

1. Preheat your oven to 350°F (175°C) and line a baking sheet with parchment paper.
2. In a bowl, combine rolled oats, almond flour, raisins, applesauce, sweetener, cinnamon, and vanilla extract.
3. Mix until the ingredients are well incorporated.
4. Drop spoonfuls of dough onto the baking sheet.
5. Bake for 12-15 minutes or until the cookies are lightly golden.
6. Let them cool before enjoying.

Avocado Chocolate Mousse

Ingredients:

- 2 ripe avocados
- 1/4 cup unsweetened cocoa powder
- 1/4 cup sweetener (stevia or erythritol)
- 1/2 teaspoon vanilla extract
- Pinch of salt

Instructions:

1. Scoop the flesh of the avocados into a blender or food processor.
2. Add cocoa powder, sweetener, vanilla extract, and a pinch of salt.
3. Blend until smooth and creamy.
4. Refrigerate for a couple of hours before serving.

Pumpkin Pie Chia Pudding

Ingredients:

- 2 tablespoons chia seeds
- 1/2 cup unsweetened almond milk
- 1/4 cup pumpkin puree
- 1/4 teaspoon pumpkin pie spice
- 1/4 cup sweetener (stevia or erythritol)

Instructions:

1. In a jar, combine chia seeds, almond milk, pumpkin puree, pumpkin pie spice, and sweetener.
2. Stir well.
3. Refrigerate for a few hours or overnight until the pudding thickens.

4. Top with a dollop of Greek yogurt and a sprinkle of cinnamon before serving.

Peach Cobbler

Ingredients:

- 2 cups sliced peaches (fresh or frozen)
- 1/2 cup almond flour
- 1/4 cup coconut flour
- 1/4 cup sweetener (stevia or erythritol)
- 1/4 cup unsweetened almond milk
- 1 teaspoon baking powder
- 1/2 teaspoon cinnamon

Instructions:

1. Preheat your oven to 350°F (175°C) and grease a baking dish.
2. Place the sliced peaches in the baking dish.
3. In a separate bowl, combine almond flour, coconut flour, sweetener, almond milk, baking powder, and cinnamon.
4. Mix until it forms a crumbly texture.
5. Sprinkle the mixture over the peaches.

6. Bake for 25-30 minutes or until the topping is golden brown.

7. Serve warm with a dollop of Greek yogurt.

Berry Crisp

Ingredients:

- 2 cups mixed berries (strawberries, blueberries, raspberries)
- 1/4 cup almond flour
- 1/4 cup rolled oats
- 1/4 cup chopped pecans
- 1/4 cup sweetener (stevia or erythritol)
- 1/4 teaspoon cinnamon
- 2 tablespoons melted coconut oil

Instructions:

1. Preheat your oven to 350°F (175°C).
2. Place the mixed berries in a baking dish.
3. In a bowl, combine almond flour, rolled oats, chopped pecans, sweetener, cinnamon, and melted coconut oil.
4. Sprinkle the mixture evenly over the berries.

5. Bake for 20-25 minutes or until the topping is crisp.

6. Allow it to cool slightly before serving.

Rice Pudding with Stevia

Ingredients:

- 1/2 cup cooked brown rice
- 1 cup unsweetened almond milk
- 1/4 teaspoon vanilla extract
- 1/4 teaspoon ground cinnamon
- 1/4 teaspoon sweetener (stevia or erythritol)

Instructions:

1. In a saucepan, combine cooked brown rice and almond milk.

2. Cook over low heat, stirring frequently, until it thickens.

3. Stir in vanilla extract, ground cinnamon, and sweetener.

4. Cook for a few more minutes until well combined.

5. Serve warm or chilled.

Tiramisu Cups

Ingredients:

- 2 cups brewed decaffeinated coffee, cooled
- 8 ounces mascarpone cheese
- 1/4 cup sweetener (stevia or erythritol)
- 1 teaspoon vanilla extract
- 16 ladyfingers (sugar-free if available)
- Unsweetened cocoa powder for dusting

Instructions:

1. In a bowl, combine mascarpone cheese, sweetener, and vanilla extract.
2. Dip ladyfingers in brewed coffee and layer them in serving cups.
3. Add a layer of the mascarpone mixture.
4. Repeat the layers.
5. Dust the top with unsweetened cocoa powder.
6. Refrigerate for a few hours before serving.

Orange Sorbet

Ingredients:

- 4 oranges, juiced
- Zest of 1 orange
- 1/4 cup sweetener (stevia or erythritol)
- 1/4 cup water

Instructions:

1. In a saucepan, heat water and sweetener until it dissolves.
2. Allow it to cool, then mix in orange juice and zest.
3. Pour the mixture into an ice cream maker and churn according to the manufacturer's instructions.
4. Transfer to a container and freeze until firm.
5. Scoop and enjoy this refreshing treat.

Chocolate Protein Balls

Ingredients:

- 1 cup chocolate protein powder
- 1/2 cup almond butter
- 1/4 cup unsweetened cocoa powder

- 1/4 cup sweetener (stevia or erythritol)
- 1/4 cup almond milk
- 1/4 cup chopped nuts (your choice)

Instructions:

1. In a bowl, combine chocolate protein powder, almond butter, cocoa powder, sweetener, almond milk, and chopped nuts.
2. Mix until the mixture is well blended.
3. Roll the mixture into small balls.
4. Refrigerate for a few hours before enjoying.

CONCLUSION

As we conclude our exploration, it's vital to remember that managing diabetes and nurturing kidney health is a lifelong commitment. It's not just about the recipes but about making informed choices daily. So, let's wrap up with some key takeaways and guidance for your ongoing culinary adventure:

1. **Mindful Eating**: Continue to be mindful of your food choices. Pay attention to portion sizes, balance your macronutrients, and savor each bite.

2. **Regular Monitoring**: Stay in touch with your healthcare provider. Regular check-ups and tests will keep you informed about your health status and guide your dietary decisions.

3. **Physical Activity**: Don't forget the importance of staying active. Regular exercise complements your diet in managing diabetes and promoting kidney well-being.

4. **Support System**: Seek support from your friends and family. Share your journey with them and let them be a part of your quest for a healthier lifestyle.

5. **Variety is the Spice of Life:** Keep experimenting with flavors, ingredients, and recipes. Variety ensures that your meals stay exciting and enjoyable.

6. **Patience and Positivity:** Managing diabetes and kidney health can be challenging, but with patience and a positive attitude, you can navigate these waters successfully.

7. **Personalization:** Remember that your journey is unique. What works for one person may not work for another. Customize your meal plan to suit your specific needs.

8. **Lifelong Learning**: Stay curious and open to new knowledge. The world of nutrition and healthcare is always evolving. Stay informed and adapt your habits accordingly.

It's time to step out of these pages and into your kitchen. Armed with knowledge, delicious recipes, and the determination to prioritize your health, you're well-prepared to continue this voyage. This chapter isn't the end; it's a stepping stone towards a future filled with wholesome, diabetes-friendly kidney meals and vibrant well-being. Cheers to your health and happiness!